Hand sanitizer:

a DIY complete guide for homemade anti-viral and anti-bacterial disinfectant

By Sam Mickelsen

Copyright © 2020 by Sam Mickelsen

Table of contents

Hand sanitizer:	1
a DIY complete guide for homemade anti-viral and anti-bacterial disinfectant	1
Introduction	4
The formulations recommended by the WHO	6
Guide to developing at the local level	6
How to prepare it? Recipe for 10 liters	8
Preparation step by step	9
On quality control	10
General information	10
Preparation area	11
Advantages of alcohol-based hand disinfection in health care	11
Information on alcohol-based antibacterial hand sanitizers, according to the WHO	12
Efficiency	13
Hand disinfection for hygienic purposes	13
Pre-surgical hand preparation	13
Lessons learned worldwide	14
The composition of alcohol-based formulations for local production	14
Unprocessed materials	14

Acquisition of components, lessons learned globally based on producer experience	16
Production and storage	17
About the production facilities and personnel	17
Storage volumes	18
Cleaning and disinfection process of the bottles	18
Quality control	19
Distribution	20
Security standards	20
Accidental ingestion	21
Conclusion	22

Introduction

There is no doubt that we live in a world that is becoming increasingly polluted and viral diseases are wreaking more havoc every day. To illustrate, the great disease of 2020 that crippled the world.
This is because we are increasingly exposed to bacteria, which are easily acquired through daily contact with people with whom we share our daily lives.
It happens at home, in the office, at school, on the street, on the bus, everywhere we spend our time.
When we are exposed to this contamination, it is impossible to avoid being carriers of bacteria, but it is possible to keep ourselves safe and try to counteract them, hence the importance of using an antibacterial gel: a practical, antiseptic and useful way without using water for our hands.
Its proven disinfectant and antiseptic action, helps to eliminate 99.9% of normal microorganisms from the hands, which means that it protects from viral diseases.
The best thing is that using the right antibacterial does not affect the environment. The gel is practical and easy to use. Just apply it to the palm of your hand, spread it over the entire surface with your fingertips and finally let it dry without shaking your hands.
Of course, health agencies recommend washing your hands often, more so these days, with soap and water, after going to the bathroom, after going out, before eating and after blowing your nose, coughing or sneezing.
Hand washing should last at least 30 seconds, and the soap should cover the palms of the hands, the backs of the hands and between the fingers, especially the thumb.
Hand sanitizers are said to be used when soap and water are not available for cleaning.

As for hand sanitizers, you have surely seen many models and sizes, colours, shapes, smells and characteristics, but not all of them are as effective or not all of them are designed to meet certain parameters, which is why in this small book or guide we will talk to you about the hand sanitizer recommended by the WHO, as well as how to prepare, store and process it. The World Health Organization recommends two types of antibacterial with very clear specifications, which are outlined below.

☐

The World Health Organization (WHO) has given many advices nowadays where the situation forces to take measures at home in order not to end up infected.
One of those advices has been the use of hand sanitizers. As expected, they became scarce worldwide just days after the pandemic broke out, where everyone has accumulated the precious product because of the situation that is unfolding.
That is why the WHO shared two formulas to be able to make hand sanitizer at home.
Before you go on to read how they are prepared, you should be careful with the indications, because if you make them in the wrong way, you can cause skin allergies when you apply the product.
Many of the homemade recipes use a mixture of two-thirds 91 or 99% alcohol with one-third aloe vera gel. The problem is that it is very difficult to control the way the alcohol is diluted in the final product, and also to ensure that the mixture does not become contaminated with bacteria.
So, in order to prepare it successfully, you must follow these instructions.

The formulations recommended by the WHO

The following guide is for the local production of hand sanitizer formulations and is divided into two specific sections:

Part A

It has indications for the preparation of the formula by pharmacists. The recommendation is that you place the information at hand so that no steps are lost.

Part B

This is a summary of the basic technical information. It is taken from the WHO Guidelines on hand hygiene in health care 2009.
There you will find important information on safety and costs, as well as information on dispensers and distribution.

Guide to developing at the local level

These are the necessary materials:

Reagents for the first hand sanitizer:

- Ethanol 96%.
- Glycerol 98%.
- Hydrogen peroxide 3%.

- Sterile distilled water and if you don't have, cold boiled water.

Reagents for the second hand sanitizer

- Isopropyl alcohol 99.8%.
- Hydrogen peroxide 3%.
- Glycerol 98%.
- Sterile distilled water or cold boiled water.

It will also be needed for both preparations:
- 10-litre glass or plastic bottles with inner screw cap.
- 50 liter plastic tanks, which are made of polypropylene or high density polyethylene and translucent, so that the level of the liquid can be seen.
- 80 to 100 liter stainless steel tanks to make the formulations without overflowing.
- Wood, plastic or metal mixers.
- Test tubes and measuring jugs.
- Plastic or metal funnel.
- 100-milliliter plastic bottles with leak-proof caps.
- 500-milliliter glass bottles with screw caps.
- An alcoholometer, temperature scale at the bottom and ethanol concentrations in v/v and w/w percentages at the top.

Of course, you don't have to have them all, these are the optional containers you can use according to the volume you are going to prepare.

As a note, glycerol is used as a moisturizer although it is possible to use other emollients for skin care. As long as they are inexpensive, easily available and miscible in water and alcohol and do not increase toxicity or encourage allergies.

Hydrogen peroxide is used to deactivate bacterial spores contaminating the solution and is not an active substance for hand antisepsis.

Any other additive added to either preparation must be properly labelled and must be non-toxic if accidentally consumed.

A dye can be added to differentiate fluids as long as it does not increase toxicity. It is not recommended to add perfumes or dyes, to avoid allergic reactions.

How to prepare it? Recipe for 10 liters

They can be prepared in 10 liter glass bottles with an inner screw cap.

What you'll need for the first hand sanitizer

- Ethanol 96%, quantity 8333 ml.
- Hydrogen peroxide 3%, quantity 417 ml.
- Glycerol 98%, quantity 145 ml.

What you will need for the second hand sanitizer

- Isopropyl alcohol 99.8%, quantity 7515 ml.

- Hydrogen peroxide 3%, quantity 417 ml.
- Glycerol 98%, quantity 145 ml.

Preparation step by step

Begin by pouring the alcohol as it comes out in the formula, put it in the large bottle or container chosen, up to the graduated mark.
Now add the hydrogen peroxide with the test tube.
The next step is to add the glycerol with a test tube. Glycerol is viscous and adheres to the walls of the test tube, so clean it with sterile distilled or boiled water before pouring the contents into the bottle.
Fill the bottle or reservoir to ten litres with distilled or boiled water. As soon as you do this, proceed to cap it quickly to avoid evaporation.
Mix everything slowly, using a mixer.
Proceed to immediately distribute the solution between the final containers. For example, half-liter or 100-milliliter plastic bottles.
The idea is that you prepare the whole mixture and then distribute it in the volumes in which you are going to use it.
Put the bottles through a 72-hour quarantine before you start using them.
During that time the spores present in the alcohol or in the new or reused bottles will be destroyed.
The final products will be as follows:

Hand sanitizer 1

- Ethanol 80% v/v
- Glycerol at 1.45% v/v.

- Hydrogen peroxide 0125% v/v.

Hand sanitizer 2

- Alcohol isopropílico al 75 % v/v.
- Glicerol al 1.45% v/v.
- Peróxido de hidrogeno al 0125% v/v.

On quality control

It is important that you carry out an analysis when there is no certificate of analysis to guarantee the tritration of the alcohol in local production. The alcohol concentration should be checked with the alcoholometer and the volume adjusted to achieve the expected concentration.

Post-processing analysis is required when working with ethanol or isopropanol solution. The alcoholometer should be used to check the alcohol concentration in the final solution. Acceptable limits should be set around +5% of the desired concentration. 78-85% in the case of ethanol.

The alcoholmeter must be used with ethanol. If used to control an alcohol solution, a 75% solution will be indicated at 77% on the scale at 25° C.

General information

The labelling used has to be in accordance with national guidelines and should reflect this information.
- Name of the institution.

- The WHO recommended formulation for hand disinfection.
- For external use.
- Avoid contact with eyes.
- Keep out of reach of children.
- Production date and batch number.
- The form of use, which states that a quantity should be poured into the palm of the hand, spread over the entire surface of both hands and rubbed dry.
- The composition of ethanol, alcohol, glycerol and hydrogen peroxide.
- Talk about how flammable it can be.

Preparation area

The best places to prepare solutions are in air-conditioned or cooled spaces. Do not start fires or make smoke. Don't even smoke.
Do not prepare more than 50 liters at a time, this because of the ventilation conditions that are not specialized, no matter how fresh the place is, it is not suitable for high productions.
Undiluted ethanol is flammable and can burn at temperatures as low as 10° C. so it should be diluted as explained above.

Advantages of alcohol-based hand disinfection in health care

It is extremely necessary to do hand disinfection to eliminate any harmful microorganisms on your hands.

Disinfection according to the WHO is recommended for these reasons:
- The rapid and broad-spectrum microbicidal activity has great advantages and the risk of generating resistance to microbial agents is minimal.
- These hand sanitizers are valuable in remote places where there are no good conditions to wash yourself.
- It promotes more frequent hand hygiene, is faster, more convenient and also saves a lot of money on hand cleaning.
- It reduces the risk of adverse effects, is safer and better tolerated than other products.

Information on alcohol-based antibacterial hand sanitizers, according to the WHO

In view of what is happening in the world these days and the effectiveness these products are showing, the WHO recommends using alcohol-based hand sanitizers for regular antisepsis of the hands.

When buying products for disinfection, it is necessary to acquire those that have in their compositions elements that understand them as effective microbicides and are accepted by health professionals. If the original compositions are seen, they will differ from the formula described above, the one described is recommended when the appropriate commercial product is not available or is too expensive.

Efficiency

These recommended formulations for hand disinfection are as effective for hygienic antisepsis as they are for pre-surgical cleaning.

Hand disinfection for hygienic purposes

The microbicidal activity of the two gels has been tested in WHO reference laboratories according to EN 1500 standards. It was concluded that the activity was equivalent to that of the reference substance, 60% v/v isopropanol for antisepsis for hygienic purposes.

Pre-surgical hand preparation

The two formulations expressed above have been tested in reference laboratories in different European countries for the purpose of assessing suitability for pre-surgical preparation according to the European standard EN 12791 although formulation I did not pass the test in either laboratory and formulation II did so in only one of them.
These recommended formulations have excellent tolerability, are well accepted by practitioners and are low cost. WHO experts state that both formulations are ideal for pre-surgical preparation.
Institutions choosing to use them should ensure that they make a minimum of three applications or more within a three to five minute period for surgical procedures lasting more than two hours.

Surgeons should then perform a second treatment with a one-minute rub, although this aspect is still under investigation.

Lessons learned worldwide

Many professionals around the world have successfully undertaken the local production of the two formulations recommended by WHO.

The composition of alcohol-based formulations for local production

The possible components of the products recommended by the WHO for hand disinfection, combine cost limitations with microbiological efficacy. Purchases of ingredients will depend on the availability of lower quality material on the market.
This is why it is important to carefully select suppliers at the local level, for preparation on site or in a locally produced facility, both formulations are recommended, as mentioned above up to a maximum of 50 litres.

Unprocessed materials

Although alcohol is the active component of the formulations, some aspects related to other components must be respected.
All raw materials, preferably used free of viable bacterial spores. In the information below you can see the raw materials that will be used in consideration:

H2O2

The low concentration of H2O2 is intended to help eliminate contaminating spores in large solutions and containers. It is not an active substance for hand antisepsis.
H2O2 adds a valuable safety aspect, although the use of concentrations of 3 to 5% for processing could be complicated by the corrosive nature and difficulty of obtaining it in some countries.
Research is still needed to assess the availability of H2O2 in different countries, as well as the possibility of using a primary solution with a lower concentration.

Glycerol and other moisturizers or emollients

Glycerol is added for the moisturizing effects to improve the acceptability of the product.
Other moisturizers or emollients can be used for skin care, as long as they are affordable, locally available, water and alcohol miscible, non-toxic and hypoallergenic.
Glycerol has been chosen as a safe and low-cost substance. Consideration may be given to reducing the percentage of glycerol in order to make the product less sticky.

Using the right water

The best would be to use sterile distilled water for the formulations, you can also use cold natural boiled water. It should not show any visible particles.

Incorporation of other additives

It is recommended that no ingredients other than those specified here be used. If they are added, the reasons for this must be justified. As well as having documentation on the safety and compatibility with the other ingredients, indicating the relevant details on the label.

There are no data available to assess the suitability of adding binders to WHO-recommended liquid formulations, as this could increase the difficulty as well as the cost of production and also reduce their antimicrobial capacity.

As already mentioned, the addition of perfumes to avoid allergic reactions is not recommended.

Acquisition of components, lessons learned globally based on producer experience

Ethanol

Given the costs, it is more viable to acquire the necessary elements for preparation locally.
It can be obtained from sugar cane or wheat.
It is conditioned by the existence of licenses and the obligation to maintain a register with several standards. It is important to take this into account for your production.

Isopropopil

It is less complex to acquire in some countries.

Hydrogen peroxide

In five places the complexity to be able to acquire it forced to import it.

Production and storage

The manufacture of the formulations recommended by the WHO for hand disinfection is possible if local governments and relevant authorities are aware of the quality controls. This will help keep production costs as low as possible.
Special rules should apply to the production and storage of the formulations, as well as to the storage of the materials. It should be noted that undiluted ethanol is highly flammable, and can burn at very low temperatures. Then it would be good to dilute it in concentrations as indicated above.
This aspect is so serious that the WHO has considered drawing up additional guidelines on scale production.

About the production facilities and personnel

The main producers of the hand sanitizers are the qualified pharmacists, of course, there are those who make them on a small scale for personal consumption.
Those who make large quantities reach good numbers ranging from 10 to 600 thousand liters per month in the test facilities.
They do it mainly in hospital pharmacies or in national pharmaceutical companies and to be able to do it they put in place the recommended containers or stainless steel and glass.

Finally they leave them in containers of 100, 385 and 500 milliliters, depending on the type of use they are going to give it.

Those who provide these containers can sometimes be a problem, because it is necessary to look for the supplier, although others have found suppliers who have provided the quantity and with the corresponding characteristics.

Storage volumes

There are special conditions regarding the quantity, conditions and forms of storage. What has been produced locally should not exceed the 50 litres stored. Even less if local or national laws require it.

Cleaning and disinfection process of the bottles

This point is extremely important, read carefully:

Empty bottles must be collected at a central location, to be treated by means of standardized working protocols.

The bottles must be thoroughly washed with detergent and running water to remove any residual elements.

If the bottles are heat-resistant, they should be disinfected by boiling them in water. This thermal disinfection is better than chemical disinfection, as cleaning with soap and other elements can be more expensive at high production levels.

If you do chemical disinfection, it is based on washing the bottles in a solution that has 1000 ppm of chlorine for fifteen minutes or more, then rinsing them with sterile or boiled water.

After thermal or chemical disinfection, allow the bottles to dry completely by placing them upside down on a suitable shelf, then cover them and store them safe from dust until you are ready to use them.

Quality control

If concentrated alcohol is obtained through local processing, the alcohol concentration must be checked, making the appropriate volume adjustments. An alcoholometer should be used to check the alcohol concentration in the final solution. The H_2O_2 concentration can be measured by volumetry, an even stricter control can be made by gas chromatography using the volumetric method to control the alcohol content and the hydrogen peroxide, respectively. In addition, the absence of microbial contamination with its spores can be verified by filtering.

Lessons on quality control

Method

The producers defend themselves by using local breathalyzers.
Seven producers sent samples to university hospitals in Geneva, Switzerland, for quality checks using gas chromatography and volumetric methods to monitor alcohol and hydrogen peroxide content.
High quality was achieved with three formulations incorporating a special fragrance or moisturizers into the WHO formulation.

Regarding climate, some samples from Mali, which had been stored in a tropical climate and without air conditioning or special ventilation, were in conformity with the optimal quality parameters, in all samples up to 19 months after processing.

Distribution

To avoid contamination by spore-generating organisms, it would be preferable to use disposable bottles, although the use of sterilizable and reusable bottles could reduce costs.
Containers of maximum 500 milliliters should be available to avoid evaporation. Containers should be leak-proof and have capacities of less than 100 milliliters for distribution to health professionals, although it should be noted that the use of such products should be limited to health care.
The production or filling unit must comply with standards of cleaning and disinfection of the bottles, such as boiling, chemical disinfection, disposable bottles should not be refilled until the product present has been completely used and the container is disinfected.

Security standards

As far as skin care is concerned, disinfecting hands with alcohol-based products is better tolerated than doing it with soap and water. Any product used to clean hands should be as non-toxic as possible so that it meets the established parameters.
As for the safety of the product, special care must be taken with it, because there is a danger of it catching fire and therefore care must be taken at all times when processing it.

Ignition temperatures

Ignition temperatures with alcohol and ethanol are 17.5°C and 19°C in hot climates. That is why it is so strict that only a maximum of 50 litres is manufactured and of course it is forbidden to generate flames nearby or smoke.

Accidental ingestion

It is unlikely that someone will consume the product, but if you are in an area with children or people who consume it, it is recommended that substances such as methyl ethyl ketone or denatonium benzoate be added to products so that they taste unpleasant and are not consumed at least in large quantities. Of course, this is for exceptional cases, because the unpleasant taste could remain in the hands and be passed on to the food without counting the fact that this increases the production costs.

Conclusion

As you can see, there are two types of hand sanitizers recommended by the WHO, which have been tested by them and have very clear specifications to be followed to the letter. Although spoken in a technical language, giving details of the production for those who want to do it massively for hospitals, laboratories or sales, it is also possible to do it locally.

Of course, as long as the health and safety measures for doing so are met.

The guide described is very clear, it shows the necessary elements and their percentage, which must be followed to comply with what is sought.

It talks about how to prepare ten-liter recipes, which can be adapted with a simple equation, to the number you want to reach.

After explaining all that is required and the care with which it is done, the step-by-step preparation is taken, which is important not only for safety, but also for the quality of the final product.

We talk about the advantages of disinfecting your hands from time to time, the preparation of these according to what is needed, from having them clean for the time being, to disinfecting them for surgical purposes.

The present guide has content for ordinary people who do not have technical knowledge about chemistry, to the most prepared doctors who know about medicine and chemistry.

Then, having in your hands the way to make good antibacterials, there is no more than to gather the elements and start doing it, remember that the quality will always depend on the care you take in its preparation.

www.ingramcontent.com/pod-product-compliance
Lightning Source LLC
Chambersburg PA
CBHW050329220526
45465CB00005B/2199